12

POSITIVE BIRTH STORIES.

By: Kiki Porter Wolff BA.RGN.RSCN.RM .

INTRODUCTION:

I have been nursing for a very long time! 21 years in England and now for 14 years in Asia. During that time I have used my qualifications in different ways. In England as a hospital nurse looking after children, special care babies, a night sister and midwife. I have run my own business from home teaching antenatal classes, maternity nursing and done some British Red Cross work. In Asia I have done freelance doula work in Malaysia, worked as a health educator at an international school in Yokohama Japan and I am currently working as a maternity liaison, medical-doula and HypnoBirthing® practitioner in Singapore.

As well as all of the above I have a fabulous husband and 2 beautiful, smart, funny daughters aged 21 and 17. I gave birth to both of them in England in NHS hospitals. It was a very different and less extravagant experience from having a baby here in Singapore.

This book will give you only positive birth stories. Why do our friends and family try and tell us the most frightening birth stories as soon as they know we are pregnant? It doesn't matter which country I am working in the people are the same. I am sure that they don't mean to be alarmists.

Not all the birth stories follow the birth plans written by the couples. Some had to have medical intervention. But they were all happy events that I was privileged to be part of, as their 'doula'.

PREPARATION for labour birth and parenting is very important. *Knowledge breeds confidence.* I have been using that phrase since teaching private antenatal classes in the mid 1980's. And it is still true today.

Kiki Porter Wolff. March 2012.

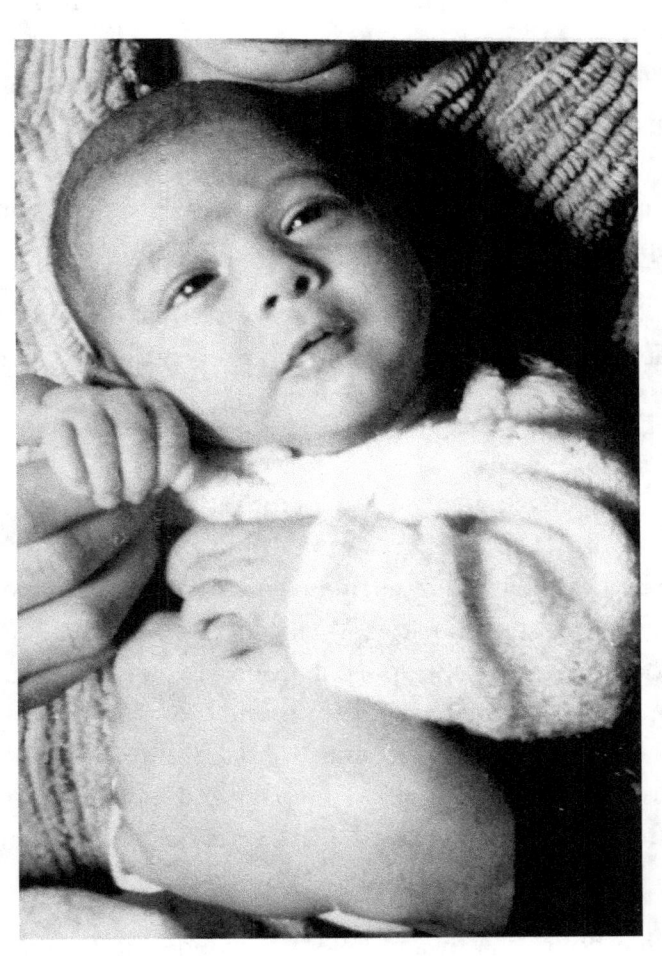

A simple birth.

I felt a little sacred and very excited, it was finally happening. My contractions started at about 2 o'clock in the morning with small period cramps that lasted a few seconds, I turned onto my side and amazingly went back to sleep. When I woke at 9am they were still there. For the next 24 hours they continued without any change and I got quite used to ignoring them. It was not until the middle of the 2nd night that they started to get stronger and longer. When I got up for breakfast and started to move around they seemed much stronger, I had to stop and breathe slowly with each contraction.

We planned to stay at home for as long as we could. By lunch time the contractions were more regular timed at every 5 minutes, I had none of the 'show' that we had been told to look out for so we assumed that I was not ready to go to the hospital yet.

The contractions continued to get a lot longer and stronger all afternoon. By the time Peter got home from work at 7pm I had had lots of the bloody show, and was finding it hard to concentrate on anything but the next contraction. We headed towards the hospital. In the car I took a pillow and wrapped it around my tummy to muffle the contractions, it worked very well and I found the hour-long journey went by quickly. We were taken straight up the labour ward and routine observations were done on the baby and me before I was free to get off the bed and walk around. My cervix was already 4cms open, I was definitely in active labour, and I was quit relieved!

The next few hours flew by and Peter was wonderful. He made sure I drank, looked after the music and made sure I was able to zone out and concentrate on the contractions without being disturbed. The next time I was given a vaginal examination I was 8cm open. It was midnight and we were getting tired, we dimmed the lights and tried to rest.

After an hour it became clear that rest was not possible, I felt as if I needed to sit on the birthing stool to get comfortable. I felt heavy pressure on my bottom, as if I had to have a bowel movement. Quite suddenly I felt a popping sensation in my uterus and warm gushing water, my membrane had broken. Clear fluid was leaking out everywhere, I could feel the baby drop, I wanted desperately to push all at the same time.

Peter rang the bell frantically and the nurses came to examine me. The examination confirmed that I was 10 cm open and ready to push. The Pushing was very empowering, it felt so good but it was very hard work. After about an hour of pushing they told me the head was close to crowning. Just then my Doctor came dashing in wearing large white wellington boots. He told me to push hard this time so I pushed with all my might. It took only another 5 minutes before our daughter was born and put straight onto my chest for a cuddle. Our beautiful little Lucy was born at 02.35 in the morning and weighed 3.0Kgms.

I had to have quite a lot of stitches but I didn't feel a thing. I was far too focused on Lucy. My labour had been slow and steady and I coped very well without any drugs. It was just as we hoped it would be. We were overwhelmed with love for our little girl.

Mary Peter and Lucy Goodwin.2010.

Medical notes:

- It is quite normal for early labour to take a long time before the body gets into a good rhythm and uses the contractions effectively. Once you reach 3-4cm of dilatation then you are in 'Active-labour'.

- Early labour can be managed at home if you are comfortable. It may depend on the distance you live from the hospital. Here in Singapore everyone drives 20 -30 min to get to the hospitals.

- Relaxation is the key to labour. Don't fight your contractions but instead LET GO and let your birthing body take over. When it is your first baby you are always surprised by the intensity of the contractions, the key is to deepen your relaxation and visualization so that your body stays relaxed and doesn't try and fight the contractions.

- Mary had me as her doula to keep her informed and to give her positive encouragement but if you don't have one the nursing staff on the labour ward will be there to look after you.

- Your body has a natural expulsive reflex that will aid the birth of the baby. When you push with your contractions you feel empowered.

1

- Here the hospital although busy has group nursing care, so that in any one labour you may have 4+ nurses looking after you all at once. You always feel well supported.

- Pain relief was available to Mary at any time throughout her labour but she didn't need it.

NB; It is always good to be open to change when going into labour. Until it begins one cannot see what the outcome will be.

Two days early.

I woke up in the morning at 8 o'clock and as I got out of bed my waters broke. Clear liquid ran down my legs and went all over the floor. Luckily we had learnt about this in our Antenatal classes so were not phased. My due date was in 2 days time! After a long hot shower I rang the hospital and as I was not having any contractions and the water was clear they told me to stay at home until the contractions begun.

It wasn't until after lunch that the first small contractions started. They felt like period pains and were short and spaced out. I decided that to check my bag was packed. The contractions carried on all day but I hardly noticed them after a while. At 6pm I rang James at work to find out how much longer he was going to be and told him I had been having contractions all day, he agreed to come home as soon as he could so we could have a meal together. After dinner the contractions felt closer together and longer but were still just period cramps, we settled down to watch a film and then have an early night. The hospital had explained to me that if my contractions still hadn't started by the morning I had to go into the hospital to prevent infection.

At 3am I felt a huge contraction and had a lot of the bloody show. It was time for us to go into the hospital. On arrival the nurses were all very calm and we quickly settled into the birthing room. I was only 3 cm open so they suggested we turn out the lights and try to sleep for a while. I couldn't rest because the contractions felt too strong. I decided to potter about the room and I coped with the contractions by sitting on the exercise ball, or standing with my hips rotating clockwise. I think I actually fell asleep on the ball for a few minutes in-between my contractions.

Our Dr came in to see us at about 6am and checked to see how much father I was open. I was 7cms. I felt very tired but hearing this news really boosted my morale and I knew that I could keep going without having any pain relief. I focused on the thought that we were going to be holding our baby in a few more hours. Those last couple of hours were a complete blur. I was coping with very strong contractions I could feel the pressure increase as the contractions pulled open my cervix. And then quite suddenly it was gone, with the next contraction I found myself wanting to push down into my bottom.

We rang the bell and the nurses came in and checked to see if I was fully open and ready to start pushing. I was. I decided to stand up using the bed for support. The urge to push down was very strong. I held my breath and pushed down for a silent count of 10 then changed my breath. I remembered from the Antenatal classes that it is very important to get 3 pushes into each contraction to keep the baby's head moving along. This was much harder than I imagined it would be.

I became exhausted pushing very quickly. I tried to imagine the baby's head coming down with each push, but it got more and more difficult. Finally after an hour of pushing I was making progress. I could see the baby's head moving when I pushed by looking in a mirror. Our Dr was gowned and ready to receive the baby and was giving me some direction. It took just 2 more pushes before the baby was born. Our Dr put her warm little body onto my chest .she felt so soft, but looked very blue, after a few seconds she started to go pink. James cut the umbilical cord and then our Dr stitched up 2 very small tears that had happened when I pushed the head out.

Proud parents James and Mandy have a beautiful daughter Ava. Our Dr was wonderful and the nursing staff all made us both feels very special.

Mandy, James and Ava Gardener.2011.

Medical notes:

- Spontaneous Rupture of the Membranes happens in only 15% of women. 50% of these women will start having contractions naturally by themselves and the other 50% will need some help to start having contractions.

- 85% of women will still have their membranes intact when labour begins. In most cases they rupture spontaneously as labour progresses but occasionally with fast or precipitate labours the baby is born still surrounded by the amniotic sac.

- The important thing to look for when your membranes have released is the colour of the water (amniotic fluid) that is coming out. It should be clear not green, red, black or foul smelling. If there is any doubt in your mind, ring the hospital to check that all is well. Some hospitals like you to ring in and report anyway.

- From 36 weeks it is a good idea to protect your mattress with a waterproof sheet just in case your membranes rupture in the middle of the night and ruin your mattress. It is difficult to wash them satisfactorily.

- After the membranes have ruptured you may have between 12- 24 hours before you have to report to the hospital if you have not started having contractions, this will depend on individual Dr's and the individual hospital protocols.

- Mandy was surprised by the amount of water loss when the membranes ruptured and it kept on leaking every time she moved until her daughter was actually born.

HypnoBirthing®. Our first.

Our baby was born on his due date! (One of the 5% that are) During our last 10 weeks of pregnancy we had been learning the techniques of HypnoBirthing. My husband Andrew and I practiced every evening, more at weekends. We had honed our technique down to a fine art. I was could relax at the drop of a hat and felt very confident that when the 'surges' started I was prepared.

The surges started at 4pm one afternoon and were short, 10 minutes apart and felt like period cramps. I didn't need to start using my HypnoBirthing®(HB) techniques at the time but they changed in nature 2 hours later, becoming much more intense. My immediate reaction was excitement. I rang Andrew at the office and told him, he bought take away food home for supper! We both felt very relaxed all evening. I took a long bath and then had an early night. I used the HB slow breathing to help me get to sleep.

At 6am I noticed some show, the surges were still 10 minutes apart but were lasting much longer. I pottered about the house, when the surges got stronger at midday I had to sit down and do some HB quick relaxation techniques. By Teatime the surges were 3 minutes apart, long and strong, I found it hard to focus on anything else, we decided it was time to go to the hospital.

When we got into our labour room I put on the Rainbow Relaxation CD and got myself relaxed before   they did the internal examination and when the nurse checked I was almost completely open. I felt so pleased with myself. It spurred me on to relax even more. I felt sleepy and comfortable as the pressure and tightening increased and my cervix opened the last little bit. Just 1 hour after arriving at the hospital I was fully open and ready to push.

We told the nurse that we wanted to breathe the baby down for a while instead of pushing. As the baby was fine we were allowed to go ahead. I got onto the birthing stool with Andrew behind me and followed my body's urge to breath down and nudge the baby slowly and gently until the nurse told me she could see the head sitting right there in between surges so she went to get our Dr.

I started using the HB J-shaped pushing technique we learned in class, it really started working. With only 3 pushes and the head was out then the body. Our son was born at 6.03pm. Holding him in my arms felt like the most natural thing in the world. He was alert and calm, and went to my breast easily within a few minutes of his birth.

Janice, Andrew and Hugo 2010.

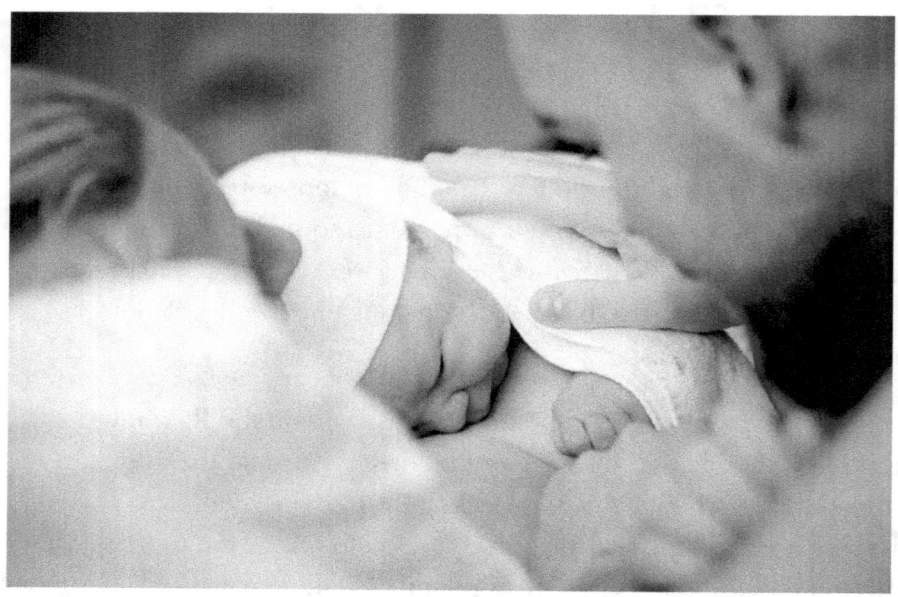

Medical Notes:

- The Marie Mongan method of HypnoBirthing® is taught in 4 or 5 places in Singapore. It is a philosophy as well as techniques of deep relaxation, breathing and visualisation that are used to manage your labour and birth.

- The couples learn the techniques during the 5-week course and have to practice together every day to perfect the techniques. Without practice they will not be successful in using the skills.

- During the labour the Mother-to-be relaxes as deeply as she can and LETS GO of the pain until her entire body is 'floppy'.

- Janice found that the stronger the contraction the deeper her relaxation had to be. She enjoyed the feeling of ultimate relaxation once she has achieved it.

- The benefits of using HyonoBirthing® include having more energy, and shorter labour. It can take less time for the cervix to thin and open. This happens when your body uses your contractions effectively instead of fighting itself.

- Her baby had the benefit of his mum practicing HypnoBirthing® throughout her pregnancy so he was used to relaxing along with her. **HB** babies are very chilled and they use crying effectively.

- The relaxation techniques can be applied to breastfeeding as well.

HypnoBirthing®. In under 4 hours.

Our first birth took nearly 24 hours and didn't go to the birth plan at all so this time we decided to take the HypnoBirthing® classes to try and make sure we had the kind of birth we wanted. My husband Jeff was really good at getting me to relax and having had surges for so many hours with my first labour I knew exactly what I was going to feel and felt that I was prepared to let my body relax totally.

My fist surge was after lunch and was short, followed by another one 3 minutes later. I felt mild pressure and tightening but felt calm and happy so I took my son to jungle gym with a group of friends. They all seemed concerned because my contractions were close together but I felt they were too short to be serious. But by late afternoon with their constant nagging they persuaded me it was time to go to the hospital. My husband Jeff met me at home and we went straight in.

During the journey to the hospital my surges became much stronger. I started using my quick relaxation technique and this helped a lot. When the nurse examined me I was surprised to find out that I was almost fully open. I was just getting settled when my doula arrived. As she walked past my bed my membranes released and splashed her down the front of her top. It was very funny because she looked so startled. We all laughed and that helped relieve the pressure I was feeling.

After that my surges then got really long and strong I had to really focus on letting my body go floppy and going to my special place in nature to cope with the sensations, but I still felt calm. A few minutes later I felt a very strong urge to 'do a poo' and lots of pressure in my bottom. We rang the bell for the nurses. They helped me get onto the birthing stool but I wasn't comfortable so instead I kneeled on the floor on a squishy mat.

My doula helped by getting me to open my eyes and look into hers whilst listening to her voice. As I did that I was able to relax and focus and 2 pushes later the head was out. My Dr almost missed it.

I felt energised this birth was so much better than my first. I was in control it was under 4 hours as I had asked for during my practice. The HypnoBirthing® really worked.

Sarah, Jeff, Alain and Leo.2011

Medical notes:

- When doing the HypnoBirthing® course the couples are asked to decide how long their labour and birth will be. Most pick 6 hours or under as the ideal amount of time to be in labour. If your body is working very efficiently labour can be short and easy.

- The visualization helps them to get into the right frame of mind. Time is distorted during labour, 20 minutes feels like 5 minutes. Relaxation and visualisation help you to let your birthing body take over.

- A second labour will usually be faster and easier than the first. Your body has muscle and cell memory that is activated with the 2nd labour.

- The newborn if well, is usually put straight onto the mothers or fathers chest for skin-to skin contact so that they can start bonding. Sarah put her son to her breast to feed a few minutes after birth. She had the benefit of experience this time and felt comfortable handling her baby.

- A first time mother may feel inept handling her newborn baby to begin with but will gain confidence day by day. A new mother will gradually learn what each of her baby's cry's mean.

- HypnoBirthing® is another tool on your belt of things to use for pain relief during labour. In my classes about 75% of the couples use it as their only tool.

Thankfully there is always Gas and Air.

When I found out that I was pregnant I was living in Singapore, it was frightening to be away from my home and family, but by the time I was ready to go into labour I felt relaxed and confident about the labour and birth of our first baby thanks to all the staff at the clinic. The clinic midwife always had time for my questions and gave me her hand phone number to call her whenever I wanted to chat.

We had a written birth plan and had been to antenatal classes in preparation, but in the end it was doing relaxation exercises that helped me to feel calm and confident in my abilities to go with the flow and let the labour unfold in its own way. My labour began with short contractions in the early evening. I felt a trickle of excitement but didn't say anything to my husband George in case it was a false alarm. The contractions carried on overnight, and in the early morning when I got up to pass urine I noticed the first bit of the show. It was just as the books described it! The contractions felt a bit longer but no stronger as I got up and went to breakfast. George had a busy day at the office so I kept quiet.

I had just finished my lunch when I stood up and had very strong contraction that took my breath away. Not sure what to do I decided to wait and see if it was a fluke or if another would follow. It did 5 minutes later. I rang George at the office. He got home in record time and began to rush around collecting things we needed to take to the hospital. We decided to go to the hospital before rush-hour traffic set in. The car ride was very bumpy and it was all I could do not to cry out in pain when the contractions coincided with the bumps in the road.

They kept us waiting for a while in the hospital but finally we got into the delivery room on the labour ward. I was very sore and stiff when trying to move on and off the bed. My examination showed that I was 5 cm open. Half way. I was feeling ok and wanted to carry on for as long as I could without any pain-relief. Thankfully I was mobile, I could walk around the room or sit on the birthing ball to rotate my hips, this helped move the contraction thorough my body. They were still 3-5 minutes apart, time vanished in the sense that we didn't notice how much time passed. We had a routine, George gave me sips of water after every contraction and I relaxed and breathed slowly through each one. My doula gave me encouragement with positive affirmations, I found listening to her voice soothing and was able to relax more quickly.

When the nurses next checked I was 8 cm open. But I knew that I was getting tired. My doula suggested using gas and air to help with the contractions from now on. The gas smelt funny but when I took in a deep breath for a few seconds I felt better. I didn't want to let go of the mask and clung onto it for dear life. More time went by; George went down for some supper and my doula stayed with me while I sucked on the gas and air. My contractions were so close together, the pressure was constant, I kept on using the gas and air to manage my contractions.

My waters broke quite suddenly with a popping sensation, warm clear liquid gushed all over the floor and over the birthing ball. Then the next contraction was huge, I took a big breath of gas and air and then had to moan because it felt so strong.

It felt natural to get onto the bed. On the bed the sensations were manageable, I felt clam again and able to focus. With each new contraction now there was pressure on my rectum. I knew I was nearly ready to push. The sensation of pressure turned into a need to push, I couldn't stop myself.

The nurses confirmed that I was fully open to 10 cm and ready to start pushing. I asked the nurses to guide me through the pushing to make sure I was doing it correctly. I was told to take a deep breath, hold it and push down for a silent count of 10, then release the breath, take another, and do it again and again until I had given 3 long, hard pushes. It was much harder than it seemed. I felt exhausted after only a few pushes. I couldn't use the gas and air while I was holding my breath to push but didn't need it any more really as pushing made me feel better. With George egging me on I pushed and pushed and after nearly 1.5 hours of pushing the midwife came to help me with some perineal stretching. I pushed for another half an hour before I could feel the baby's head in my girly bits. I couldn't tell exactly where she was but it felt full and heavy, as If I was sunburnt down there.

The Dr came in and got everything ready and I felt a rush of adrenalin that gave me a surge of energy. It took another 6 pushes before the head was crowning, then her body was out. Tears of joy were streaming down my face. George was crying too. We were so happy to see our little baby girl looking normal and healthy.

The rest was quit a whirl of activity. The placenta was delivered a small tear was stitched up. I barely heard what the Dr was saying to us as I gazed at our baby. Looking back I am happy with the way the labour went. It was 12 hours in total and went smoothly. I could not have done it without my doula's knowledge and encouragement.

Karen, George and Ella. 2010.

Medical notes:

- Gas and Air is a mixture of 50% Nitrous Oxide and 50% Air or Oxygen gas. It numbs the pain centres in the brain and also dulls the pain messages being sent by the brain. It works without making you sleepy or unconscious. The mixture is called Entonox.

- To use Entonox, wait until the start of a contraction, then inhale slowly and deeply through your nose using either a facemask or mouthpiece to activate the flow valve and release the gas, then exhale slowly. AFTER 2/3 breaths you will notice the pain relief and a feeling of wellbeing. Continue to inhale until the contraction has gone.

- Karen stopped using the gas in between contractions because it made her feel disorientated and sick. Not everyone feels like this. Entonox crosses the placental barrier but is eliminated from your body and the baby's body rapidly causing NO harmful effects.

- You can't breathe in the gas and air while holding your breath to push so doesn't use it during the 2nd stage if labour. However it can be used as pain relief while the Dr sews up any tears if you need it.

About 55% of labouring women find they manage just using Gas and Air as pain relief.

Entanox can work well with different relaxation techniques to add a little extra help relaxing if needed.

I loved my epidural.

Our birth plan looked wonderful, it had everything we wanted for our completely natural birth. We knew that it was just a plan and that things didn't always go as planned, but that wouldn't happen to us.

Labour started as expected with mild cramping below my pubic bone. The contractions were very short and 10 minutes apart. I didn't ring Hugo immediately because I wanted to make sure it was not going to turn out to be false labour. By the time I had re-packed my bag, done the shopping cooked and eaten lunch they were still coming every 10 minutes and felt about the same. I was sure that I was in labour and rang Hugo. He came home and we spent the afternoon looking at each other wondering if it was time to go to the hospital yet. We rang the hospital, they told us to stay at home until the contractions were 5 minutes apart, lasting over 60 seconds.

By 10pm they were finally 5 minutes apart, feeling stronger. They still didn't hurt so we thought we should try and sleep. Hugo was asleep in seconds but I just dosed on and off in between the contractions. By 5 o'clock in the morning I felt exhausted and wanted to go to the hospital for support. We missed the rush hour traffic so got there quickly. When the nurse examined me I was 3 centimetres open. I was disappointed, but there was nothing to do but relax and let my body do what it was supposed to do naturally. We tried the birthing ball, the floor mat, sitting in the chair, walking around the ward and finally lying in the bath for a few hours each but I didn't make much progress. By 2pm I was still only 4-5 cm open and I was feeling very frustrated. I felt as if I was doing something wrong.

It was then that my doula suggested that I wasn't relaxing deeply enough, I was fighting the contractions. In my heart of hearts I knew that she was right. I looked outwardly relaxed and calm with each contraction but inside I was struggling with each one. When I felt one coming it took all my powers of concentration to appear calm and breathe slowly through it. I didn't want to let Hugo down by using pain relief but I knew couldn't go on much longer without any progress. When I told him this he was very supportive and we all decided I should have an epidural.

The anaesthetist was lovely and made me feel much better about my decision. It wasn't painful to have put in because he chatted to me all the time he was doing it. After a few minutes I felt the pain of the contractions lessen. The nurses turned me onto each side, onto my back, to make sure that the pain relief worked evenly on both sides. The effect of the epidural was amazing. After hours of trying to cope with the contractions I felt myself again. The contractions were still coming every 5 minutes but I could not feel them at all. My legs were very numb and difficult to move around but I could feel the baby move inside me which was reassuring.

Our doula suggested that Both Hugo and I snooze for a couple of hours. So we settled down and actually managed to sleep while she stayed with us reading her Kindle. When the nurse came to check me I was 8 cm open, and 2 hours after that I was fully open and ready to start pushing. The down side of my epidural was that I was so numb I couldn't feel any pressure as the baby's head came down or the urge to push with my contractions. The nurses had to tell me exactly when and how to push and I had to try and do it without any feeling. But I slowly began to make progress.

After nearly 2 hours of exhausting pushing the head was visible and ready for crowning and our Dr arrived. With his encouragement I managed to push effectively, the baby was born a few minutes later and put straight onto my chest for skin-to-skin contact and bonding.

The flood of emotion I felt was overwhelming and I found myself crying as I looked at my son's beautiful face. Hugo cut the cord and then the Dr stitched up a large tear. I had been a very frightened of the pushing stage because friends had got me worked up about it telling me horror stories. But with the epidural I felt as if I was in control. Thank god for the epidural.

Katie Hugo and Harry 2010.

Medical notes:

- Having a doula with you doesn't stop you from having an epidural if you need one. She will stay with you throughout your labour. In fact women who plan to labour without pain relief and then turn to epidural often feel disappointed in themselves and need more support not less.

- Katie felt disappointed she had resorted to an Epidural, but she enjoyed the birth so felt that made up for it in the end.

- A birth plan is just that 'A Plan' of how you wish your labour and birth to go. Obviously there may be unseen factors that may affect your stamina on the day of labour, or special circumstances that arise during the labour and you will have to adapt. The safety of your baby is most important.

- An Epidural is a regional anaesthetic and in most cases removes all the pain, but this also means that you cannot feel the urge to push when the time comes and this makes pushing more of a challenge.

- Everything is left on the table when it comes to labour and pain relief. You always have the choice to have help if you need it.

I always stay with my couples throughout the entire labour and birth, anywhere from 4-48 hours. It is a privilege to be asked to attend a couple's birth as their doula.

3rd Time Lucky.

I can't thank my doula enough for all her guidance and kindness. Without her our baby would have been born by caesarean. We had had 2 easy labour and births in the past and never considered that the 3rd one would be any different.

My waters broke as I got out of bed one morning 2 days before my due date. The water was clear and continued gushing for about 5 minutes. Afterwards, every time I moved I felt trickling down my legs, but no contractions. The hospital told us that we could stay at home for 24 hours before coming in unless the contractions started to get strong before then. They didn't start at all. So we went in the next day for induction.

According to the Dr my cervix was ready and he felt that just a tablet would do the trick and start labour. The put it in at about 8am and I stayed on bed rest for an hour of monitoring before being allowed to get up and walk around. Nothing had happened 4 hours later, our Dr wanted to put up a drip to get labour going. We were disappointed, we asked if we could try another tablet first but he said that my cervix was soft already and it would be less tiring if we started the synthetic oxytocin, so much for our natural labour. Still there was nothing we could do so we tried to be cheerful. I could still walk around with the drip. The contractions started immediately and were gentle at first. The nurses adjusted the drip until the contractions were every2- 3 minutes apart. These felt different from the natural contractions I had in the past. Perhaps it was all in my mind I am not sure, I was anxious and found it harder to relax and breathe through the contractions, which were now stronger.

The next few hours went quickly, I was just able to cope with the contractions but knew that I was getting to my limit. I needed to have to have an epidural this time. We asked the nurse to set it up for us, the Dr Came to put it in half an hour later. The odd thing is that while waiting for the Dr to arrive my tolerance for the pain dropped to almost nothing, it was as if I had already given up.   My doula and my husband Ross had to work very hard to stop me from losing control. I managed, but when the epidural was in, it was bliss. I went back to being my normal self.

My cervix opened quickly after the epidural was put in, I was fully open and ready to push in 2 hours but the baby's head was still very high so my doula suggested breathing down the baby for a while instead of pushing straight away. I did this by relaxing and not holding my breath when I had the urge to push. My epidural was turned down so that its affect would wear off so that I could feel some pressure with the contractions.

Another 2 hours later and the baby's head had moved down but it was still too high. There were signs that baby was beginning to get tired because his heart rate was dropping at the wrong time and the Dr gave me 2 choices. Either I had a caesarean section in the next half an hour or he could help me to have a vaginal birth using the vacuum.

 I was terrified I completely lost it and started sobbing. Ross didn't know what to do, the nurse was talking about caesarean, and it was my doula that managed to calm us down by gently going through both options from our baby's point of view. After a while I could talk again and Ross and I agreed to have the vacuum birth the Dr offered if it was still safe for our baby. While I practiced pushing the Dr got his suction cup ready and put it onto the baby's head. Then with the next contraction he pulled while I pushed and the head started to come down. A few minutes later I had my baby out and in y arms. She was beautiful even with a small cone head. They put her onto my chest and I held her very close to me breathing in the unique newborn sent. We had done it, a girl and 2 boys. I had no episiotomy and only a small graze so no need for stitches.

We both felt elated. Despite having the epidural, the vacuum the birth went well, we felt positive about the experience. After 2 'natural births this was different but in no way a bad experience. Thankfully we are in a country that offered us all the choices and had a **VERY GOOD DR.**

Alice Ross James Harry and Lucy.2011.

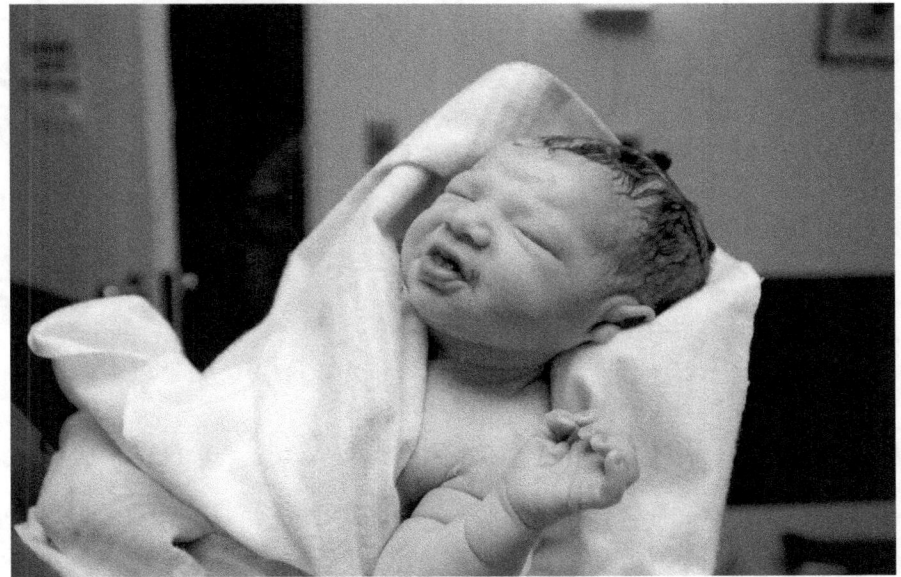

. Medical notes:

- If the baby's head can't descend enough on its own to come through the birth path and the baby and mother show signs of fatigue. Your Dr may then suggest that he helps you with an assisted delivery. This is usually vacuum or forceps to help deliver the baby while you push.

- You will need an epidural or spinal block to have this procedure, as it can be painful without any pain relief. This allows you to have a vaginal birth, rather than a Caesarean birth.

- Babies born with vacuum assistance have a scalp swelling called a chignon; this looks like a small cone and will vanish in a few days with no lasting effects.

- Alice got very tired pushing by herself. She saved the rest of her energy to help the Dr with the vacuum. She didn't need any stitches afterwards because she has already had 2 vaginal births without tearing her perineum the 1st and 2nd times.

- Some Dr's would not have offered her the choice but gone straight for the caesarean section but her DR was very experienced and knew that it was safe for both mother and baby.

We tried everything!

During the Antenatal classes we learnt about natural labour without using any drugs, with drugs as well as inductions, and having a C-section but felt smug in the knowledge that we wanted was an easy labour and birth. We ended up using everything in the book.

Labour started as the book said it would with mild contractions in the evening. I went to bed and woke the next morning with stronger contractions 3 minutes apart and some show, so rang the hospital. They told me to make my way in for a check. When we arrived they hooked me up to the machine that reads the contractions and the baby's heart rate, I was having good contractions. My cervix was 4 cm open already I was staying in hospital. Time went by quickly, a light lunch was served, and the contractions seemed to be getting stronger. At around 2pm our Dr came to check on me and I was more open. The labour was going slowly but steadily. Jeff was in good spirits and was looking after me beautifully, making sure I had sips of water every half an hour and offering me snacks to keep my energy levels up.

At 5pm the Dr came back again and checked me but I was still at the same point I was 3 hours before, my labour had stopped. He offered us the option of having the water bag popped to try and speed things up, and we agreed. It was a bit sore but I was ok. The water was clear (healthy) so we were left for another hour to see if it made a difference. By 6.30pm I was having very strong contractions but had only improved by half a centimetre. The Dr suggested I have an epidural to help me relax for a while and see if labour would progress on its own.

The epidural was wonderful; almost as soon as it was put in the pain from the contractions stopped but left me shaking uncontrollably for a few hours while my body adjusted. My head was clear again and I found that I could relax, even doze. The contractions got much stronger while I relaxed but didn't feel anything, and started to open my cervix again. By 7.30pm I was almost fully open and ready to push. My legs were varying degrees of numb and I could not feel any sensation of wanting to push so they turned down the epidural. The nurse told me not to worry she would instruct me what to do when the time came.

However by 9pm my cervix still had not fully opened. The baby's head was still high and his heart rate was being affected. Our Dr decided that the baby would have to be delivered in the next hour or two at the most. We all agreed to give it another hour to see if I could fully open and start pushing.

10pm arrived, I was finally fully open but the baby's heart rate was dropping alarmingly. They asked me to breath in oxygen using a facemask to help the baby's heart rate pick up, which it did thankfully, the midwifes were flapping around and all looked so serious that it make us very frightened. When our Dr came back into the room he was fabulous, he took one look at the graph from the machine and then said, don't worry, you are going to have your baby now. He was so confident and so clam that we didn't feel frightened any longer. I was whisked off to the operating theatre, the epidural was topped up to maximum and they swung into action. Fifteen minutes later I was holding my son and he was perfect.

The cord was wrapped once around our son's neck and was also very short which was why he wasn't happy once he started moving down the birth path so his heart rate dropped. The Dr' and our medical-doula were both very calm and efficient which made us feel safe. It all happened so fast in the end that we didn't have time to stop and think.

Our son's birth may not have gone according to our birth plan, but it was always *positive* and the medial care we got was excellent. Having tried everything this time if we have another baby our birth plan for the next birth will be less ambitious.

Andria, Geoff and Sam. 2011.

Medical notes:

- Eating and drinking in labour are very important to maintain the mother's energy levels. Approximately 100 calories per an hour during labour are required in the form of energy bars and juice boxes etc. Nibble and sip! Don't try and eat a 3 course meal when you are in labour your body can't digest all of that!

- Vomiting during labour is quite normal. Many women vomit nearing or during the 2nd stage and after delivery.

- Occasionally labours become very long and complicated. If problems develop your Dr will have to make a decision quickly that offers the safest choice. In this case it was a caesarean section.

- Andria trusted her Dr and was happy for him to decide what to do to keep their baby safe.

- In a real emergency the baby can be born almost immediately, but usually they have about 30 minutes to arrange a caesarean and get you ready for theatre.

- Having a spinal block or Epidural for a caesarean section means that you are awake and will see your baby being born.

I am too posh to push!

From the moment we knew we were going to have a baby we decided that Caesarean section was the best way for us to have the baby. I have 4 sisters all of whom have had babies in a variety of ways, none of which appealed to me at all. We wanted to pick the date of the baby's birth and didn't want to have the uncertainty of not knowing when and if we were in labour, followed by the long hours of labour, which may or may not go according to plan. NO the quick, planned birth was for us.

So it was the day I was 38 weeks that we arrived in the hospital at 6 am to have our baby. We were very excited, about to be parents and eager to get going with the operation. The formalities took about half an hour and then we were left alone in our room to wait, and wait. At about 7.30am the nurse came to take us into the operating theatre. I felt nervous about the procedure it was very cold in the corridor waiting to go in which made me more nervous. After a while the nurses gave John an all-in-one-sterile suit to wear over his hair and clothes, shoe covers and mask. I was in a gown and also had a hat covering my hair.

The staff got me onto the operating table and connected me up to bits of equipment. The anaesthetist chatted to me as he started to put in the spinal injection that would make me numb. He put an intravenous tube into my hand so that he could hydrate me and give me something to help me to relax, which was great. The nurses put a barrier up in front of me so I couldn't see what was happening on the other side of it. My Dr tested to see if I could feel any pain before he started the procedure, I couldn't but I could feel tugging. It took about 15 minutes until our baby arrived.

Our Dr held up the baby for me to see before he gave her to the paediatrician who checked her out from head to toe and then gave her to me to hold for a few minutes.

Her little nose was pressed up to mine it was difficult to see her features because there wasn't much room to move because only my arms were free. She felt wonderful. After a few minutes in my arms she went to John, he and the baby went out to weigh her first then to take her up to the ward to keep her warm. I must have slept for a while because when I woke they were transferring me onto a trolley and taking me out of the operating theatre. The whole thing had taken less than an hour. Back on the ward, John greeted me holding our beautiful daughter Millie in his arms. We cried with joy and hugged her close all day.

My recovery was fast. I spent the day of her birth in bed waiting for the spinal to wear off and my body to get back on track. The day after the birth they took off all the equipment and I was encouraged to get up slowly and potter about. Wearing the corset really helped with getting in and out of bed and moving in general. By day 2 after the birth I was up and about, had showered and was able to breast feed in the chair.

We were very happy with our choice of birth for Millie. My bikini line scar healed quickly and I felt rested after having to take it easy for 6 weeks. My breastfeeding went very well and we have never looked back. I will do the same next time.

Mary and Millie 2010.

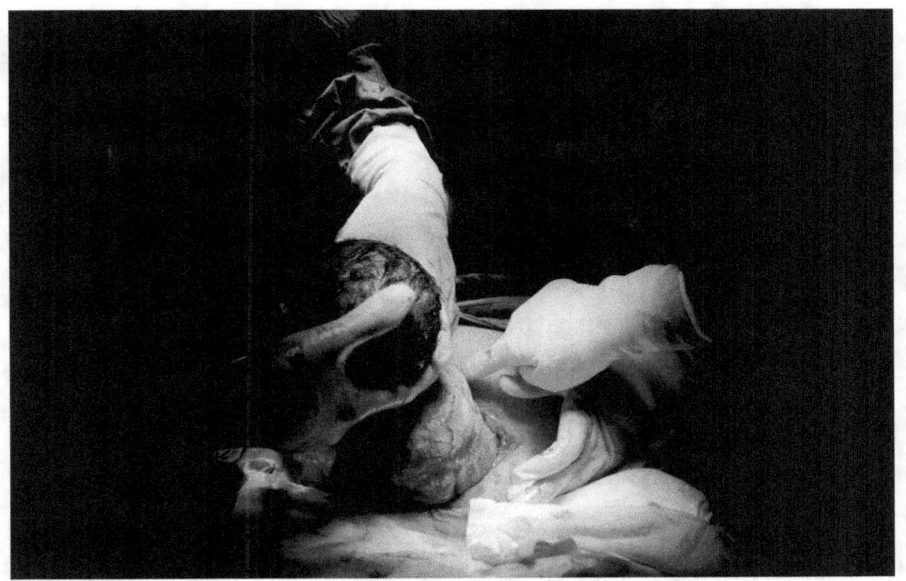

Medical notes:

• It is every woman's right to choose the way she wants to give birth to her baby. There are many reasons why a woman could choose not to go through a vaginal birth. For example: Some people have attended a birth and have been put off by it. Others have had a bad experience that they don't wish to repeat.

• If your baby lies bottom down instead of head down then this is called a Breech position. Most Dr's feel that caesarean is the safest way to deliver your breech baby. There are websites that can give you things to try to turn your baby into the cephalic position (head down) they involve hanging off the sofa upside down and various other positions as well as relaxation and visualization. Some women feel that they must try everything to turn the baby into the correct position for a natural birth. Others are more philosophical about it.

The baby doesn't stay cuddling with mum in the operating theatre during a caesarean for more than a few minutes after its birth because they keep the theatres cool and the baby looses its body heat very quickly. Dad and baby will go up to the postnatal ward together to bond with skin-skin contact (if the baby is well) while they wait for Mum.

In Singapore we put wraps onto women who have had caesareans to keep the wound supported while it heals. This allows you sleep well because you can turn more easily in bed and when walking it doesn't feel unsupported.

Most women benefit from the 6 weeks of forced inactivity giving them rest, time to come to grips with breastfeeding and a good supply of milk.

We had our 2nd Baby in Singapore.

My aim was always to have as natural a birth as possible. I had used the HypnoBirthing® method for the birth of my first child in the UK, but this time, away from home and in Singapore, I wanted more support for the birth and chose to have a doula be there with us as well as using HypnoBirthing® again.

A couple of days before my due date I felt very ready to have my baby. He had been in the right position for several weeks, I had done lots of HypnoBirthing® practice and everything at home was ready for the baby's arrival, even my hospital bag was packed. I went to the reflexology place that I had been going to regularly throughout my pregnancy for a foot massage and asked the therapist to push the points that are thought to bring on labour. Three hours later I had my show, an hour after that my waters broke. At this point I had no contractions and so, after a quick chat with my doula over the telephone, I went to bed to get some rest.

The next morning I woke up with mild contractions about 10 minutes apart. I stayed in bed and slept until I noticed that the contractions were becoming stronger and closer together, we decided it was time to go to the hospital. We arrived at the hospital and were met by our doula at around 1pm. All the birthing rooms were full so we were put into a holding pattern in the waiting ward. I was measured at nearly 5cms dilated. The breathing and visualisation exercises I had practiced were really useful for the next couple of hours while we stayed in this waiting area. Our doula really put is at ease we were in safe hands. The affirmations I had been listening to during my HypnoBirthing® practice repeated in my head as the contractions grew stronger, and they really helped me to relax.

It was not until 3pm that we were shown into our private birthing room. We settled in, setting up our relaxing music, cracking open the lunchbox size juice cartons and snacks. I lay on the bed and continued to relax, using the affirmations, breathing and visualisation exercises throughout each contraction and then just resting in-between them. It made all the difference to have our private room. I found that I could focus much more quickly.

At 5pm I decided to I wanted to know how dilated I was. I had that feeling of fullness in my bottom that told me I must be nearly fully diluted. My doula called the nurse to check me who told me I was 8 cm dilated. I felt a bit disappointed, I still had 2 cm to go, I was hoping the birth would be a quick one. Trying not to be discouraged I asked my husband and my doula if we could start some of the relaxation exercises and the light touch massage we had practiced in the hope of speeding things up at bit. It worked. My son was born less than an hour later at 6pm. It was an indescribably joyous occasion, I will never forget the sense of achievement I felt for giving birth to my son naturally. We had skin-to- skin contact straight away and started breastfeeding in the first hour of his life.

I was up and walking around just a couple of hours after giving birth, in no pain other than a few post-labour pains when breastfeeding and mild backache. We were able to spend our time in the hospital resting and getting to know our new baby without anything detracting from our enjoyment of this special time. I feel very privileged to have achieved the natural birth that I wanted and thankful for all the benefits that have come with it.

Sasha, Matt & Eddie. Singapore.2011.

Medical notes:

- Having a baby is a foreign country is often daunting. You don't have your usual support network of family and friends to lean on. Having a doula attend your birth is a good way to feel supported.

- Happily HypnoBirthing® is taught in Singapore so Sasha felt that she could use the same skills she had used for her first birth. This felt familiar. I gave her a few refresher classes at home to make sure that her techniques were working for her. She has her husband had practiced the techniques a lot before the birth.

- A great sense of achievement is felt when the birth does go according to plan. Sarah was in a good frame of mind while preparing for her 2nd birth.

- *Sasha was able to recognise the contractions/surges from her first labour. She noticed that her HypnoBirthing® techniques worked better the 2nd time around because she knew what to expect. She was able to get deeper into self-hypnosis and really let go allowing her birthing body to take over.

When abroad and away from home at the time of your birth surround yourself with family, friends or support people so that you don't feel you and your husband have to cope with a new baby alone.

Home Birth after all.

Our first baby was born in the UK at home as a water birth. We were hoping for something similar here in Singapore but found that there was only one doctor who did them at all and it was not our Dr of choice. Our Dr worked mainly in one hospital and never did home births. We decided that having the baby at home was not as important as having the Dr we felt comfortable with so we decided to take the HyonoBirthing® course which the hospital offered to help us get into a natural frame of mind in a hospital setting. The HypnoBirthing® practitioner agreed to be our doula during the birth, which gave us both great peace of mind. We worked hard and felt prepared when the time came.

My labour started with a feeling of pressure across my abdomen in the morning. I ignored this and had a normal day pottering about with my daughter at home. By the late afternoon the pressure had increased and moved from across my tummy to my bottom and back as well. Deciding it was time to go to the hospital I rang my doula to ask her to meet us at the hospital. As I got up to leave the house my waters broke and the baby's head started coming down very fast all at the same time. I felt anxious that I was not going to make it to the hospital.

 My husband rang our doula again. She felt that the baby was coming now and told Yannais what he should do to receive the baby and then wait for her to arrive in the hospital ambulance. By the time the call finished and he came back to me I was in a state of panic. We had not prepared ourselves for a home birth!

I was trying not to scream, I knew our daughter and her friend were in the next room and I could feel the top of the baby's head in my vagina. Yannais looked very pale but gently guided our baby out as it was born and then picked both of us up and carried us to our bed. He wrapped us both in a blanket and then sat down looking dazed. He rang our doula and told her the good news.

I was shocked, but also happy, I had another home birth, it was what I had really wanted. By the time our doula and 2 midwives arrived in the ambulance the placenta was starting to be delivered. I had put the baby to my breast straight away to keep him warm and toasty. Thinking back I believe that I ignored the feeling of pressure I had been having all day because I wanted to have my baby at home.

Ilana & Yannais 2010

Medical notes:

- In the old days Singapore used to do lots of home births, but as time has progressed fewer and fewer Dr's are doing them. Today it is quite hard to find a Dr that will let you have one because there is not flying squad back up to come to collect women who have their babies at home id needed in case of emergency. Special arrangements have to be made for a home birth in advance. It is not a good idea to decide to have one when you are in labour.

- Some women are frightened in hospitals and want to have their babies born at home where they can be relaxed and calm. Almost all births here in Singapore are in hospitals. We try and make the women feel at home by adjusting the atmosphere in the birthing rooms to make them less clinical. One hospital in particular did over 100 water births last year.

-
  Ilana wanted to repeat her lovely first home birth with her second labour and birth but couldn't have her chosen Dr if she wanted a home birth so had to change her plans. When her labour began she felt very relaxed at home and delayed going into the hospital, because of this her labour progressed much faster than she recognised and the baby was born at home by mistake (as she wished)

- HypnoBirthing® mothers don't recognise the feelings of pressure and tightening they are having in labour as pain. It is quite normal for them to find that they have progressed much further than they expected when assessed. This is because they are in a good mindset and allowing their bodies to take over their birthing.

A Water- HypnoBirithng®

Knowledge breeds confidence! That was the phrase our midwife-doula used. Well we had lots of confidence. Joss and I took 3 different antenatal courses with different companies to make sure that we had as much information as we needed. When I first found out I was pregnant I definitely wanted to have a C-section, I didn't want to feel pain and go through labour like everyone else. But by the time we had been to 3 courses I had changed my mind. I wanted a water birth, in hospital, using HypnoBirthing® techniques. Instead of using drugs to combat pain the techniques taught us deep relaxation and visualization that would empower us to 'let go" of the pain and let my body labour more efficiently.

My labour started in the middle of the night with mild surges. These lasted all day and most of the 2nd night as well. By the 2nd morning they began to feel much stronger and longer. We rang our midwife-doula who agreed it was time to go to the hospital so that we could get settled into our delivery room with the birthing pool.

By the time we arrived an hour later I was definitely having very strong surges and needed to get into the birthing pool straight away. At once the surges slowed down and gave me a break, I relaxed and floated in the pool and gradually they started up again as before. I was very comfortable, the surges were getting stronger and longer but in the pool I felt in control of my level of relaxation. I rested while my body laboured. After I had been in the pool for about 4 hours I could feel the baby moving down the birth path slowly with each surge. The midwife checked me in the water and told me that I was fully open. She told me I could breath down or push when I felt like it. I was quite happy breathing down the baby so didn't start pushing.

After a while I could feel the baby's head on my bottom. With each surge I felt him coming closer and closer. I could feel all my tissues stretching as he came down. Finally the midwife said she could see the head easily and I gave a little push with the next surge. Our son was born with 2 pushes and floated out into the warm water in the pool. When we lifted him up out of the water he took his first breath. He was clean and warm. I found that having him in the water felt very natural and we were all very relaxed and calm for his birth.

Joss. Wendy and Sam. 2011.

Medical notes:

- HypnoBirthing® and water birth combine very easily. The mind over matter required to prepare for both types of birthing techniques are similar and compliment one another.

- Joss found the water very comforting and this helped cue her HypnoBirthing® deep- relaxation techniques. Just getting into the birthing pool in not enough. Without having skills the water alone is not enough to get a woman through labour without feeling pain.

- Joss became one with the water and relaxed deeply letting go of all external distractions. While allowing her birthing body to take over completely.

- In most hospitals water births have to be booked in advance to make sure that qualified midwifery and nursing staff are on duty. In hospitals that specialise in water births this may not be so.

- Joss hired a birthing pool from her midwife. She was able to practice with it at home and had it set up in her conservatory.

- There are strict health criteria but a woman who has had a normal uneventful pregnancy can have a water birth as long as her labour progresses normally.

- Both mother and baby are relaxed and calm during a water birth.

Conclusion:

In an ideal world, every woman would feel empowered and in control during her labour and the birth of her babies and all babies would be born into a calm and gentle environment.

It is very important for pregnant women to let go of their fears about labour & birth before they go into labour themselves. Fears can manifest in labour as complications that may stall the labour or prevent the body from working efficiently. *Let go of any negative feelings* you have and focus instead on positive affirmations, stories and experiences. Prepare yourself for labour and birth. Practice relaxation techniques to make sure that you don't fight your labouring body. *And stop reading horrific things on the Internet!*

A successful *doula* is one who has learnt to listen, and has the ability to blend in with her environment. All we want is a positive birth, where the baby comes into the world gently and calmly into the arms of loving parents. All our preparation during pregnancy is make the labour and birth easy and happy and the world the baby will live in safe and nurturing.

No matter where or how you choose to give birth to your baby you can influence the outcome by taking control of your labour. *Knowledge breeds confidence.* Mind over Matter: For every thought there is a physical reaction in your body. You can influence the way your body reacts by changing the way you think about labour and birth. Practice the techniques you learn in the Antenatal classes until they become second nature. Ultimate Relaxation is the key even If you have to use an Epidural to achieve that ultimate relaxation.

I have noticed that couples that work together to manage pregnancy, labour and birth develop a special bond. The old days of fathers sitting in the waiting room handing out cigars has been replaced by proactive dads who are part of the birthing process.

A birth plan is just that, a plan. It gives you a chance to sit down and think about the things that you would like during your labour and birth. You are in control, even if it is your first labour you have a choice.
Circumstances may change during the labour and birth but you will adapt and change your plan accordingly.

I hope that after reading the positive birth stories in this book you are now feeling more excited about your own labour and birth.

Don't be afraid to ask questions from your care providers.

Kiki Porter Wolff BA.RGN.RSCN.RM March 2012.

ABOUT THE AUTHOR
KIKI PORTER WOLFF

I was born at Westminster hospital in London in 1958. My mother went into early laobur at 34 weeks of pregnancy. She knew instinctively that it was going to be fast and was rushed to the hospital by my father.

The nursing staff took their time with the admission procedure thinking that mummy was not very far along. New mothers-to-be never knew what was going on! I was born 30 minutes later just as they were getting mummy in to the bed in the observation ward on the labour floor. I weighed the same as a bag of sugar, but was strong and didn't need to go into an incubator.

My poor mother was in Westminster hospital for 12 weeks until I gained enough weight to go home. She made the best of it and looked after some of the other women, keeping them cheerful. She would tell you that my birth was a positive one.

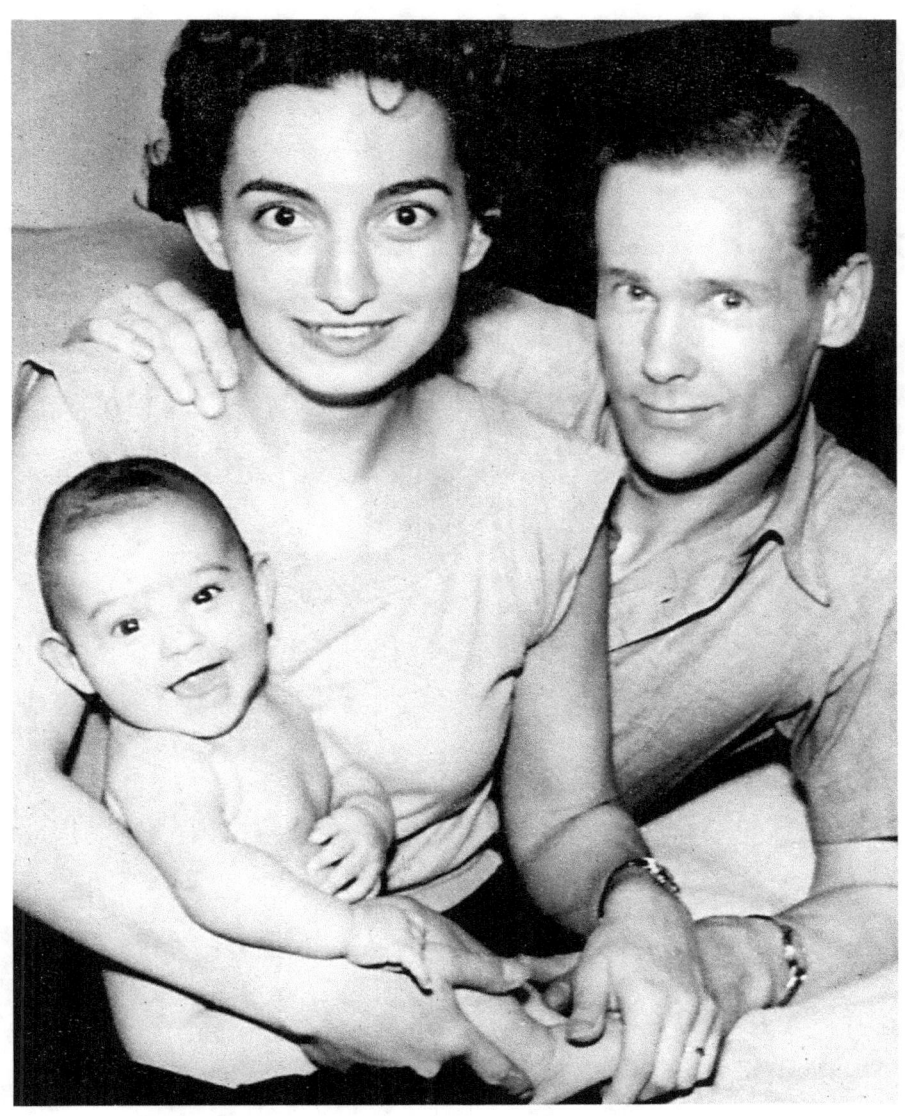

Kiki Porter Wolff in the arms of her proud parents Tina and Maurice Porter. 1958.

www.ingramcontent.com/pod-product-compliance
Lightning Source LLC
Chambersburg PA
CBHW060226290526
45789CB00003B/1427